Caseness and Narrative

Contrasting Approaches to People Psychiatrically Labelled

Michael A. Susko

AllrOneofUs Publishing
Baltimore, Md & Huntsville, Al

While every precaution has been taken in the preparation of this book, the publisher assumes no responsibility for errors or omissions, or for damages resulting from the use of the information contained herein.

CASENESS AND NARRATIVE: CONTRASTING APPROACHES TO PEOPLE PSYCHIATRICALLY LABELLED

First edition. April 22, 2020.

ISBN: 978-1393315759

Written by Michael A. Susko.

Table of Contents

This book is dedicated to those who protect rights of persons going through a variety of "lived experience."

Caseness and Narrative originally published in *The Journal of Mind and Behavior,* (Winter and Spring 1994) Volume 15. Numbers 1 and 2 Pages 87-112. Amended and edited, 3/29/2020. Published with permission from the editor of the journal.

Cover Art by NovOntos, *Pearl of Great Price*

INTRODUCTION

Recent times have been marked by a number of autobiographical narratives from psychiatric survivors, one of the most politically powerless groups in our society.[1] Because ready-made biological explanations of madness are pervasive in our society, first-person accounts offering a different viewpoint have difficulty accessing the mass media and making any sustained public impression. Such stories, from the "inside out," compel us to reexamine the traditional Caseness approach of psychiatry.

Caseness is an intellectual construct that facilitates the objectification of a person in the medical system: the person becomes a "case" or is primarily perceived as one. This article critiques the Caseness approach, which dominates the mental health system, and contrasts it with a Narrative approach. In brief, Caseness emphasizes making a diagnosis of illness and stopping its symptom expression. The Narrative approach, on the other hand, supports individuals coming to their own voice by allowing their story to unfold and to be told.

A narrative segment from *Cry of the Invisible* illustrates the basic difference between the two approaches. Joe Green tells of an incident at a state hospital:

> *Due to my excessive spiritual reading and my disorientation, I started to act out the things I had read. I would throw books on the floor and think I was waking up humanity by vibrating the spiritual energies throughout the earth. An attendant noted this. That night, another attendant took me into a seclusion room and physically wrestled me to the floor. Somebody else put a needle in my backside. They shut me up all night. (p. 198)**

Although Joe was trying to awaken humanity, he woke a few attendants instead. No one asked Joe why he was throwing books on the floor, or tried to find out what he meant by "vibrating the spiritual energies of the earth." The Caseness approach required no further explanation for Joe's behavior, having already established that he was "paranoid schizophrenic." Joe was not encouraged to communicate the meaning of his "acting out," as this might be viewed as encouraging the disease.[2] Instead, Joe learned to hide the expression of his inner thought, becoming, in effect, invisible. As he goes on to report:

> *The next morning I was more docile, frightened. This is what they wanted: orderly, behaved people, so they would only have to observe. From then on, I didn't act out because I would be thrown in seclusion and get the needle. (p. 199)*

The Caseness approach labels the unusual experience as a disease entity and seeks to maintain this label, separating the person from "normal" people. The Narrative approach, on the other hand, seeks to place the life story with its difficulties as part of a common human experience.

Until the 1860s, it was routine for the patient's own account of his or her illness to be taken by ward clerks upon admission to any hospital.[3] This practice of allowing narrative meaning was lost as medicine's attention to what was natural for the sick individual—allowing for idiosyncrasy—was supplanted by what was considered normal. Clinical practice became increasingly obsessed with comparing "measurable signs" to "standardized norms."[4] A more systematic comparison of Caseness and Narrative, using examples from experiences labeled as schizophrenic, is presented below.

* Cited in Susko, M. A. (Ed.), 1991. *Cry of the Invisible* Baltimore, Maryland: The Conservatory Press. Throughout this article, the author draws on examples from this anthology of first-person narratives that he collected and edited from several psychiatric survivors.

PART ONE
THE CASENESS APPROACH

The Caseness approach consists of three stages, which follow and reinforce each other in a circular way: 1) identifying target symptoms; 2) making a diagnosis; and 3) intervening to stop or manage symptoms. I will critically examine the assumptions underlying each stage.

I. Identifying Target Symptoms

The initial assumption is that a pathology is the sole cause of symptom expression. A hidden and more significant assumption is that the symptoms are to be negatively valued. Modern allopathic medicine does not typically pay attention to patients' interpretations of their symptoms and illnesses, much less their positive regard for them. Originally, the word illness signified what the disease meant to the patient, while disease referred to physical pathology.[5] In the book *Intoxicated by My Illness*, Broyard illustrates this view when he describes his search for the "positive metaphors of illness."[6] But generally in recent times, symptom (the person's expressed distress) has collapsed to sign, a biological marker.[7]

Other societies have not held such a restricted view. Suffering had meaning and served as an opportunity for cure and spiritual advancement. Indigenous cultures might interpret illness as a "call to enter into association with powers you are less familiar with."[8] A survey cited by Bynum found that over half of female medieval saints had illnesses that were an integral part of their sanctity.[9] In modern times homeopathic medicine has sought to enhance symptoms to affect cures.[10]

But for mainstream culture, disease, illness, chemical imbalance, and genetic defect have only a pejorative meaning. Where productivity and "survival of the fittest" are heavily valued, disabled people or those who drop out of the work force are stigmatized.[11] The concept of a "diseased mind" carries connotations that are doubly negative. Not only does it evoke disability, but it arouses fear and implies that a person is not responsible for his or her mind, or is difficult, unpredictable, and potentially violent. The net effect is a marked lowering of the individual's social status.

A second assumption in identifying symptoms is that they can be targeted, i.e., decontextualized from personal, familial, and social/historical experience. The phenomenon of "mental illness" is seen as "independent of the environment."[12] This view originates from casework, which reduces the personhood of the patient to Aa series of medical facts that ignore one's hopes, dreams and fears.[13]

In reductionist thinking, the mind is considered a function of the brain. The medical model does not consider that multiple levels of meaning can exist simultaneously, and that anyone level can dominate in a given instance. It ignores, for example, that subjective feeling can precipitate bodily changes, that after a feeling "molecules materialize."[14] A dynamic body/mind interaction can give weight to both subjective and bodily meaning. Jung held that the "more physiological" functions (such as eating and digesting) are intimately related to the "more archaic and 'deeper' symbols."[15]

Joe Green, in his narrative from *Cry of the Invisible,* stated that his problem was "due to my excessive spiritual reading and my disorientation." Prior to his hospitalization, Joe relates that he experimented in meditation practices, "high energy frequencies," as he later termed it.[16] In order to "ground himself" while in the hospital, he tried to awaken "the lower frequencies of the earth." Thus, the symptoms, in the context of Joe's story, were an attempt to find his spiritual/ physiological balance. Healing the body by making physical contact with earth energies has a long tradition among indigenous peoples, as with the Australian aborigines.[17] Thus, Joe's so-called acting out not only makes sense in the context he establishes, but in a political way, as an awakening of Western humanity at this historical time, one that seeks to make contact with the "Mother Earth" and with ecological values.

Is symptom identification placed within any meaningful biological context? Psychopharmacological texts and current essays of researchers admit that proof of physical causation of "mental illness" is lacking.[18] In a recent symposium on schizophrenia, a researcher stated that if he were captured by neuroscience terrorists and told to prove that schizophrenia was a brain disease, he "would be very hard pressed."[19] His best evidence, that 25 to 40% of first-episode patients have enlarged brain ventricles and tissue atrophy, is "a very nonspecific finding..." about which he says, "I have in no way any implication of what that might be..." In spite of such professional admissions, the disease model is offered to the public as a scientific fact.

There is no medical test, blood sample, or brain scan that can prove the presence of a "schizophrenic illness."[20] Although some patients evidence disturbance in their dopamine systems or have enlarged ventricles,[21] these signs could derive from a number of causes in any given person. The diagnosis depends on the doctor's characterization of a self-disclosure. As Thomas Szasz says, "the evidence for [schizophrenia] is still only the fact that crazy people often talk crazy."[22]

Even if there were evidence of biological differences in "schizophrenics," the Caseness approach would not be justified. In any altered or normal mental state, one would expect biological correlates.

The brain is a very plastic organ, sensitive to experience. Pert goes so far as to say that the brain's dynamic receptors "change in shape from moment to moment."[23] Trauma, severe mental distress, as well as drug treatment can cause brain alterations, even damage. But evidence for such changes does not prove that "mental illness" is primarily a dysfunctional biological event. Finally, even if "schizophrenia" were biologically based, it would not mean that "brain imbalances" warrant biological treatments. Putting a person in a more loving environment might ameliorate symptoms as effectively or more so than prescribing a course of drug or other biological treatments.

The so-called biological model of psychological distress remains a hypothesis about the relationship between certain neurotransmitters and certain behaviors. The speculative nature of biological psychiatry has led Lehrman to term it molecular phrenology.[24] Within this model, Joe Green's experience is reduced to excessive secretion of dopamine in the limbic area of the brain. Yet, despite the model's emphasis upon biology, the relevant biological context is easily missed. Many environmental toxins, illnesses, or even medical drugs can cause psychoses. Striano cites several studies reporting that from ten to 50% of patients have undetected physical illnesses that "either caused or worsened their psychiatric illness."[25]

This raises the question of what characterizes "mental disorders" and psychiatric treatment? For many, the answer is obvious: a care giver helping a distressed person. However, several forces can impinge on that ideal characterization in any given instance: the psychiatrist as an agent of control over groups that deviate from the dominant social order;[26] indigenous people with their "uncontrolled emotions";[27] the desire to suppress the cries of abused individuals;[28] the wish to keep intact dysfunctional families;[29] or a method for dealing with people who are obnoxious, an issue which the literature rarely addresses,[30] except with "difficult patients" who are often diagnosed with "borderline personality disorders."[31] Some feminists describe the concept of madness "as a means of dismissing and controlling women."[32] In a feminist analysis of the classic story, *The Yellow Wallpaper*, Treichler describes a "clash between two modes of discourse: one powerful, 'ancestral' and dominant; the other new, impertinent, and visionary."[33] Other factors that can compromise treatment include streamlining and standardization of care by insurance companies and the "managed care revolution,"[34] the "selling of clinical psychiatry" to research needs,[35] and the pharmaceutical industry and its "accustoming the physician to pharmaceutical largess."[36] In his analysis of scapegoating, Williams believes that "American culture has become a pharmacy" as a way for people to "conceal their own violence by a series of substitutions."[37]

All the factors mentioned thus far assume that some persons possess "right sense and sanity" and have the expertise to identify those outside such boundaries. These "experts" determine that certain expressions of distress reflect a biological pathology, and are not in fact related to personal, family, or larger societal concerns. The professional, with what could be termed a hyper-rational form of madness, is ready for the second step.

II. Making a Diagnosis

The basic requirement in this stage is that the diagnostic category already exists. An examination of the construct schizophrenia, however, reveals that it is a soft one.[38] Experts disagree whether the entity actually exists, whether it is a single phenomenon, or whether the diagnosis is a sort of "dust bin" collecting all types of experience.[39] In short, there is little or no consensus on what is being measured or how to measure it.[40] The title of Bentall's article illustrates the diagnostic disarray: "The Syndromes and Symptoms of Psychosis: Or Why You Can't Play 'Twenty Questions' With the Concept of Schizophrenia and Hope to Win."[41]

Professionals admit that there is no single unifying idea that can unite the phenomena of "schizophrenia."[42] Various frames of reference have been offered, including: "a disturbance of cognition"[43]; the "failure of historicity"[44]; the "experience of pure objectness"[45]; a "mystical-occult breakthrough"[46]; and Bleuler's belief that the unity and harmony of personality is being "split up."[47] A recent neurodynamic model, based on computer simulations, posits "memory parasitism" which "coercively draws" many neuronal excitation patterns into a few repetitive ones.[48]

Diagnosis may appear to be the end result of a diagnostic process, but often it frames which symptoms are noted and reinforced. Barrett shows how the diagnosis directs the clinician's attention toward early behaviors which reveal "schizoid" traits and meet the diagnostic criteria, as well as to characterize the person's life history as an "epic of failures," culminating in "schizophrenia."[49]

With naming comes a transfer of ownership of the person's mind and body to the professional. If someone's brain is diseased, that individual ceases to be viewed as a responsible owner of his or her mind/body. This logic is legally encoded in the "Not Guilty by Reason of Insanity Plea," based on the concept of "diminished responsibility." The question of ownership has not been altogether lost by some professionals, as it was raised recently in the book *Psychosurgery: Damaging the Brain to Save the Mind* with a chapter heading that asked "Whose Mind Is It Anyway?"[50]

Patients confronted with forced treatment can become very aware of the issue. A feminist woman in her 30s, who was hospitalized and forcibly drugged, tore off her hospital bracelet and told the staff, "This is my body."[51] Uncomprehending, the staff made her put it back on. Nurses and attendants, as representatives of the medical system, function as the new owners of the patient's body/mind and use invasive chemotherapy. Some patients have portrayed the hospital as a giant "influencing machine," with their internal organs hooked to it.[52]

Fuller Torrey reports a "Rumpelstiltskin effect" derived from the act of naming.[53] Because a problem is identified and named, there is said to follow a therapeutic effect, by giving the person a sense of control over the problem and offering the promise of cure. But naming can also stigmatize, the word stigma suggesting a physical embeddedness in the body. "Mental illness," which holds to some sort of bodily defect, means one cannot trust his or her body or its resultant thoughts. As for social stigma, Hubbard and Wald say that history shows that "grounding difference in biology does not stem bigotry."[54] The racial hygiene movement of Nazi Germany first eliminated mental patients or "useless eaters" before using the same methods on the Jewish people.[55] Ethnic cleansing in Bosnia has reached a "neo-biological intensity," and brutalities in South Africa have constituted a type of ethnic cleansing on the "surplus," "idle," or "unassimilable."[56]

Likewise, the "mental patient" can suffer dire consequences from his or her biological label. When the realization sets in that one is vulnerable to forced treatment, that one must take powerful drugs for the rest of one's life, such that living a full life is no longer possible, and that one is caught in a "revolving door syndrome" of repeated hospitalizations, then the "Rumpelstiltskin effect" wears off and the grief sets in. Torrey does not mention what happened to Rumpelstiltskin after he was named. Brothers Grimm tell us: he "sunk into the earth" and "tore himself completely in halves."

There is evidence to suggest that those who accept the label of mental illness have a worse course in their illness than those who reject that identity.[57] Is this because medical naming reduces people and their experience to invisibility? Or does such naming lead people to vent their symptoms in yet more radical, extreme ways, making them seem even more "mentally ill?" One could argue that any person who is "freeze-framed" with an identity as a mental patient finds that identity ultimately damaging.[58] Establishing the ownership of someone else's body through diagnosis creates more helplessness or more extreme manifestations of symptoms. But whether "negative" or "positive" symptoms ensue, the aim of treatment is the same: stop and control symptom expression.

III. Intervening to Stop Symptoms

That the goal of psychiatric procedures is to control, manage, and if possible stop symptoms is suggested by the frequent use of phrases like "treating symptoms,"[59] "symptomatic improvement,"[60] and "normalizing" symptoms,[61] and is illustrated by the choice of drugs (neuroleptics such as Thorazine and Haldol) used in the front-line treatment for schizophrenia. Research using psychedelics which enhanced symptom expression was conducted in the United States at Spring Grove Hospital in the 1960s and early 1970s and recently was legalized for very limited use.[62] Early clinicians labeled the neuroleptics as "ataractics,"[63] meaning they offered freedom from confusion or anxiety, but the later label, "major tranquillizers" is a more accurate description. According to one researcher, the name was changed, once again, to "anti-psychotics" more for political than for scientific reasons.[64]

A basic, if unstated, assumption of the third step is that if a person's symptoms are stopped, his or her pain or distress will be lessened. In the 1950s researchers noted that the drugs' primary effectiveness was in reducing psychomotor agitation, the outward expression of distress. As for the inner feelings of delusions and hallucinations, H.L. Gordon cited studies that they were only partially controlled, with one quarter to one half of the people showing no improvement.[65] Contemporary researchers allow for substantial groups of people who are "non-responders."[66] As Theodora, in *Cry of the Invisible,* stated, "The drugs don't stop the pain but the scream of the pain."[67] A person confined to a psychiatric hospital could be left in the intolerable position of being in intense inner pain without the ability to physically express that pain. And if, as some models hold, hallucinations or delusions are present to distance people from their pain or traumatic memory, then symptom removal may open the floodgates to the original pain.[68] For any given person, the question needs to be raised: will control of symptoms increase or lessen pain?

One may also ask whether it is always good to stop or lessen pain. Change, any growth experience, may cause what Jung called "the suffering of individuation." Ironically, the avoidance of pain has been said to form the essential characteristic of "mental illness."[69] This avoidance of pain, the clinical focus on stopping symptom expression, may characterize the existing system. It may describe a client who avoids issues he or she needs to face, or a psychiatrist who simply increases drug dosages in response to increased distress in the patient. Indeed, the psychoanalyst Masson characterized his teachers as "shut away from these private worlds of pain."[70]

A second assumption of the last step is that treatment is symptom specific, that somehow only the undesirable expressions can be removed while the larger person remains unaffected. Yet early researchers readily compared the effects of Thorazine to those of lobotomy, in the days when lobotomy held little negative stigma.[71] That the drugs produce a global flattening affect is well established, as is the fact that they have been shown to produce a host of iatrogenic diseases.[72] Ex-patient narratives are replete with reports like the drugs make one feel like a "zombie," causes "a glass wall between us," or an elaborate description termed "reductive-reactive," that is, "I had reactions to them, and they reduced my ability to cope, by causing so many reactions."[73]

Ironically, psychotropic drugs often create behaviors that more readily identify the person as "mentally ill." Dr. Baldessarini illustrates:

> *It's very easy to confuse bradykinesia with so-called negative symptoms of schizophrenia. It's very difficult to differentiate the restlessness of akathisia from agitation in psychotic illness... You have to pinch yourself, force yourself to think differentially in every case, every day, as to whether you're overdosing and causing part of the problem that the patient is having.[74]*

Are the symptoms or is the person being stopped? And if the treatment has indeed stopped the person, is not the person "decontextualized," thus buttressing the initial assumption that the person's experience is simply biological?

A routine manifestation of the third step is pressured treatment - verbal argument, and coercion, such as threatening continued hospitalization until compliance is gained. Lucksted and Coursey found that 30 to 40% of clients in rehabilitation programs have been treated forcibly or threatened with removal of a benefit.[75] Although formally used on a minority, forced treatment has a chilling effect on the larger group. Residents come to know that, if necessary, force can be justified by an expansive definition of "danger to self or others."[76] The implicit ideology of force in psychiatry, illustrated with vocabulary such as target symptoms, intervention, and front-line worker may be said to represent the culmination of a type of "military mentality that medicine often adopts."[77]

In summary, the Caseness approach focuses on identifying symptoms that are negatively valued and assigns them a medical diagnosis. Labeling facilitates the transfer of ownership from the person to the medical system, which allows that system to use force when necessary to stop expressions of distress. The Caseness approach engenders a certain story and meaning, but it is essentially the same story for everyone who is so labeled: "I have a mental illness caused by a chemical imbalance in my brain. To control this disease, I must take medication for the rest of my life." Undergirding this is the realization that, "If I refuse treatment, force by medical people can be used against me."

PART TWO
THE NARRATIVE APPROACH

The essence of the Narrative approach is that it helps the person find meaning within the flow and context of a life story. Narrative typically has a temporal frame, a series of actions leading to a turning point or climax. This process reveals character, what in autobiography is called an "act of self-identification."[78] Narrative also has a theme or moral, what Maine terms *emplotment*, the ability to come to a point.[79] Thus, narrative differs from chronicle "as in string of biological signs" because it establishes significance to the physical sequence, one that reveals deeper structure and brings a sense of closure to the person.[80]

Here, the literary tool of narrative is offered as an alternative to Caseness for understanding and helping people labeled with mental illness. While Caseness already advances a biological meaning, Narrative tends to have no predetermined answers, and allows people to establish their own explanations. Thus, a woman who sees her problem in terms of feminist ideology should have a therapist familiar with those beliefs, one who could engage in dialogue from that frame of reference.

This paper does not offer treatment modalities making use of narrative concepts, as some psychoanalysts have already done.[81] Instead, it puts forth the assumptions necessary to reframe our orientation, out of which specific treatment modalities may develop. The Narrative approach can be examined as a three-step process: 1) allowing the story; 2) using the narrative as the frame of reference; and 3) supporting the story's transformative potential.

I. Allowing the Story

Letting the story unfold assumes a positive value for symptoms or expressions of distress. This assumption has its roots in philosophic thought from Plato's expression of "divine madness" to the Renaissance scholar Ficino, who believed that "poetic madness" could calm a soul experiencing "disorder and dissonance."[82] The medical literature holds analogous beliefs dating back at least to Pinel's *A Treatise on Insanity*, wherein he observed that some patients show "paroxysms of active insanity" that are "salutary efforts of nature to throw off the disease."[83] A minority of contemporary professionals admit potential value in "psychiatric episodes,"[84] and occasionally the literature carries titles such as Corin and Lauzon's "Positive Withdrawal and the Quest for Meaning,"[85] or Burnham's "Symbolic Vessels for Voyages of Self-cure."[86] But such views are the exception in a profession that focuses on deficits of persons labeled mentally ill.

Various approaches exist that have a positive regard for expressions of distress. One fundamental is that the "breakdown" represents a death/rebirth experience, a passage where the person "dies" to old ways of being in order to grow and become more whole.[87] Kaam and Healy believe that the theme of "recurring death and rebirth of personality" underlies world literature.[88] To illustrate, we can turn to Chretien de Troyes, the first major Romance writer of the Middle Ages. In a literary analysis of Eric and Yvain, Artin sees "Yvain's lapse into madness and his return to sanity as typologically imitative of Christ's death and resurrection."[89] In *The Brothers Karamazov*, Mochulsky believes that the three brothers represent stages in the life of Dostoevsky. Alyosha, for example, is a symbol of the writer after his imprisonment, when he experienced a "regeneration of his convictions."[90]

Indigenous rituals also embody the death and rebirth theme. Mircea Eliade described such rites in which "initiatory death is often symbolized...by darkness, by cosmic night, by the telluric womb, the hut, the belly of a monster." The individual who emerges from the ordeal has a new and different being.[91]

People undergoing "schizophrenic breaks" frequently use death and rebirth metaphors. We find a clear example, that of "melting," in Jack's Story. "Something inside me was dissolving in a way I could not stop. To control it, I usually took a cold shower, four or five times a day, or as many times as necessary."[92]

The Caseness approach holds that Jack is experiencing somatic hallucinations and is engaging in obsessive-compulsive behavior. But Jack explains the phenomenon differently:

> *[The melting] was a loosening up of tension. The body armor that had made me distant and afraid was breaking down. Usually my body and muscles were tensed, keeping my feelings guarded, and protecting me from painful feelings. The "melting," as I understood it, was not only a result of the release of subconscious feelings but a breakdown of my usual means of protecting myself from awareness outside my normal range of consciousness.[93]*

First, we note that Jack ascribes a positive value to his experience. The melting allows him access to his feelings. Jack's melting is a "dying" to his old rigid way of being and presages new life. To understand the melting phenomenon, one may turn to the archaic symbolism of water. Eliade held that water was preeminently a "killing," dissolving symbol, and thus "rich in creative seeds.[94] In a process called *solutio*, Renaissance alchemical texts speak of powerful emotions dissolving the body, and its "materialistic egotistic attitude."[95] Perhaps in modern times a person going through a crisis/life passage can experience "inner waters of dissolution." In any case, psychiatry would miss this possible interpretation due to what Kirmayer calls "a hyper-rationalism that ignores the significance of bodily felt meaning."[96]

The vulnerability of the "schizophrenic" experience offers parallels to that of indigenous youth who go through tests, including periods of isolation and fasting, in order to enter into full adult society. Initiates may act helpless like infants "re-learning to eat and walk," experience altered or visionary states, or go through symbolic wounding and dismemberment/ re-memberment.[97] In the Amazon, initiation is held to be comparable to that of crabs and other animals that shed their old shells or skins, and gain a "new skin."[98] Not only does "schizophrenia" in Western societies typically occur during young adulthood, but the individual may experience regression that mimics infancy, somatic feelings of falling apart, and states of consciousness that have been compared to the initiatory call of the shaman.[99] Combining anthropological and psychological models, Mason asks us to "re-vision clients' pathology into a desire for initiatory experience."[100] Van Gogh, perhaps the most famous artist of contemporary times, compared his periods of inner turmoil to a "molting time," where after a period one emerges renewed.[101]

Psychoanalytic attempts to understand "schizophrenia" have at times offered a death/rebirth interpretation. Pious describes the experience as an encounter with nadir, which is "figuratively a momentary death."[102] Symptomatic behavior becomes in effect a "progression from the nadir" with definable stages moving toward increased health and integration. More recent transpersonal theories hold that the struggle through various birthing stages, "perinatal matrices," serve as a gateway to the transpersonal domain, to a mystical connection with all beings.[103]

Our society generally fails to provide rituals of initiation. The turning of youth toward illegal drugs has been termed as a "disorderly and desperate expression of this need" for initiation.[104] In drug use, however, the rebirth experience precedes the death experience, where the taking of the drug is the birth and the coming down from the drug is the death. One wonders whether psychiatric drugs, insofar as they are neurotoxic and disabling, mimic a symbolic death and lead to a premature natural one. Hallstein goes so far as to say that hospital stays (for physical illness) mirror the liminal nature of initiation rites. "Lying thus stripped, isolated, pulled away from the family and community, facing possible mutilation, pain, or death, the patient is presented with the possibility of confronting the ultimate meaning of his or her existence...."[105] But one questions whether such "rites" in the mental health system, that inflict pain involuntarily and incur permanent stigma, risk being experienced as torture, an "unmaking" of the person and the destruction of his or her voice.[106]

In what could be seen as a type of death/rebirth experience, catharsis makes use of symptom expression to achieve healing. In this approach, old wounds and traumatic experiences, often going back to childhood, must be "discharged" for healing to occur.[107] Large percentages of psychiatric survivors have suffered from some form of past abuse.[108] Such traumas will naturally seek release, provided a safe setting is established. In psychoanalytic language, Bromberg and Balint describe the process as one of benign or therapeutic regression.[109] Considerable literature has developed around the phenomenon of dissociation stemming from past abuse, and the need for the fragmented self to reintegrate.[110] At times the person simply needs a proper container for his or her symptom expression. One ex-patient, who "had too much going on inside," saw her times in the hospital seclusion room as beneficial because that allowed her "to play out her story."[111]

Another metaphor for positive valuation of symptoms may be called "running to the opposites," a term used by the Greek philosopher, Heraclitus. The therapeutic notion that cures may be affected by opposites, that the induction of an opposing passion can help rid a person of a disturbing one, was further articulated in the Renaissance.[112] According to Jungian analysts, one sometimes goes to extremes to redress an imbalance. People who assume little or no responsibility in their lives may, during a breakdown, suddenly feel responsible for everything. A person shut off from inner exploration may be suddenly penetrated by "beams," exposing innermost recesses. At times, the psyche goes to the periphery of human experience so that the center can be found.

The positive regard for symptoms assumes that, in crisis, the psyche naturally moves toward healing, toward finding authentic identity. Sass suggests that those diagnosed with schizophrenia suffer from too much meaning, that they grapple "not with entities but with Being."[113] John Weir Perry describes the "psychotic process" as "the spontaneous emergence of the central archetype."[114] Alice Miller, using more everyday language, states, "My illness helped me to hear the voice of the child I once was, the voice I had tried to silence for so long."[115]

One may consider that a person suffering distress bears a privileged truth.[116] Thevoz, the curator of the Collection de l'Art Brut in Switzerland, believes that the "mad" delineate and make clear structures that are in everyone's psyche.[117] Artists such as Jackson Pollock and Lenora Carrington had breakdowns which helped them come to their distinctive art form.[118]

Symptom expression is not always transformative and healing. A Bosnian woman, who repeatedly screamed in distress, was described as "frozen in her story."[119] Symptoms may turn into a destructive spiral and possibly stop the person's life for years. There is also the danger of "the seduction of madness," feelings of specialness and "grandiosity" that could keep the individual imprisoned in a symbolic world.[120] Still, we should not mistakenly assume that symptoms are always negative.

The Narrative approach asks us to reexamine our bias against symptom expression and look at the communication inherent in it. We must ask, as Cohen did during his lifetime of clinical practice: "What are these symptoms trying to solve which the person can't solve in any other way?"[121]

Positive valuation of symptoms creates a power ambiguity. If the person is having a transformative experience, something of potential value to the individual and the society at large, that experience is something to protect and support. This was, in part, the rationale for isolating people during initiation rites; not only to protect them, but to protect society from the overflow of their spiritual energy.[122] John Weir Perry believes that the experience of "schizophrenia" can go beyond "personal individual initiation."[123] In times of cultural crisis, the individual may assume a "prophetic," "semi-revolutionary" role and become an agent of cultural change and revision. Once a doubt is raised as to the power status of the modern "mentally ill" person—the possibility of respect for what may be a life passage and/or a message for others—the way is open to use Narrative as a frame of reference.

II. Using Narrative as a Frame of Reference

Frustrated by "profound disciplinary failures," various disciplines ranging from sociology to medical anthropology are turning toward a storied approach, in what has been termed the "narrative moment."[124] In the arena of psychology and mental health, a variety of terms have emerged, including "illness identity work,"[125] "autopathography,"[126] "hysterical narrative,"[127] and "survivor discourse."[128] Such works may have their historical origin in "conversion narratives," which are "often attended by visions, hallucinations and impulses to atheism or suicide."[129] More recent "autobiographical essays," favored by existentialists, describe the experience of "dislocation," and one's coming to an identity that is "provisional" and "incomplete."[130] Change is the essential feature in these varied narrative types, the transformation of the self or one's persona[131] toward a richer, more complex direction.[132]

Narrative has the ability to convey the inherent thickness and richness of life events.[133] If the consciousness in "madness" is inherently shifting describes as "its energetic alteration, its endless metamorphosis,"[134] then narrative would be an apt tool to convey this quality. When Fleischmann writes in her journal, "Voices inside, the inescapable I ...and the heart, too, is never still,"[135] we have a much richer feel for her inner state than a clinical note such as "Pt. is restless, hearing voices."

Narrative can convey complex notions of the self. Recent anthropological views have challenged the standard assumption of "the egocentricity of the self," to one that is more dynamic and fluid.[136] Hermans, Rijks, and Kempen see the self constructed as a "polyphonic novel," with multiple voices engaged in dialogue.[137] Such a novelistic view may come closest to the "schizophrenic" experience with its shifting, "alternative frames of reference."[138]

Putting experience within the "narrative web" can lead to insight.[139] Narrative organizes the chaos of experience, establishing connections between events.[140] What might otherwise be seen as isolated and senseless symptoms of distress reveal themselves to be meaningful parts of a person's life story. In *Cry of the Invisible*, Theodora recounts that she suffered a gang rape, then was hospitalized a month or two later. At no time did the professionals ask if there had been a recent trauma, and when she finally volunteered the information to a nurse, she was not believed. Only after she told her story for publication, did it become apparent to Theodora that there was a connection between her attack and subsequent hospitalization. Through the narrative process, people come to see that earlier life events and patterns are dynamic connected and forces acting in the present.

There is a narrative *fit of truth*. An event is meaningful and true because of the way it fits into the life story.[141] We listen and read how a seemingly minor event can be the hinge on which the story moves. In *Cry of the Invisible*, Ron tells of a patient he sees "with his hands and feet turned inward" caused by the effects of neuroleptic drugs.[142] From that point, Ron's life is changed, and he becomes an advocate to fight the "bio-coercive model" of psychiatry.

Although narrative illuminates connections to past events, revealing a determinedness to events, it also casts the person as active in making decisions, even in the most seemingly determined of events. Sarbin states that it is critical for people to perceive themselves as "agents trying to solve existential and identity problems."[143] Even though Jack succumbed to coercion to take psychotropic drugs, he repeatedly heard an inner voice telling him that he was "about to make a big mistake."[144]

A sense of narrative itself is necessary to gain a moral sense, the ability to give an "account of oneself," as well as to expand our ability to perceive different sentiments.[145] In the article "When Narrative Fails," R.C. Allen holds that people can live authentic lives only when they come to emancipate themselves from a larger dominating story, or when they see how their own story is embedded in a larger one.[146]

The narrative lens helps us see the texture and connectedness of events, including the self as a dynamic agent, able to make choices. The Caseness approach, in bringing its energies to bear on making a differential diagnosis, can easily miss these elements. The point is shown explicitly in a case study that compared tape-recorded interviews to the written record. Paul Lawrence, a psychiatric patient diagnosed with schizophrenia, revealed that a friend died from a drug overdose a week before his own breakdown. Paul then makes comments like, "I can talk to him spiritually. . . . [I have] communication with the spiritually dead." Later, he reports that his friend is warning him: "Get help! Get help! Help yourself!"[147] The interviewer focused several questions on the way Paul worded this communication, trying to fit it into the criterion of an exterior voice for the schizophrenic diagnosis. Meanwhile, the fact that his friend's death is of significant concern to Paul was left unnoted in the case record, nor that Paul's experience of it could be a critical resource for his healing. This example illustrates a fundamental flaw in Caseness, its failure to bridge the divide between doctor and "patient." It has led Charon to say, "No wonder they miss one another in the dark."[148]

In telling his or her story, a person names the experience, and so establishes the discourse from which any explanation proceeds. Explanation may be framed as a search for meaning, a problem in relatedness, or as a cry of outrage against abuse or oppression. Michael 0., for example, sees his core problem as a moral crisis, his inability to make a true confession, to really tell someone what he is feeling.[149] The poet Roethke framed his "manic episode" as a mystical experience he had with nature: "Suddenly I knew how to enter into the life of everything around me. I knew how it felt to be a tree, a blade of grass, even a rabbit."[150] The naming can lead to what Emerson refers to as a "higher sort of seeing."

Not all people have the articulateness of a Roethke, and there is often a "narrative darkness,"[151] or a silence within narrative that can only suggest the inexpressible. As one writer from a Canadian collection of ex-patient stories put it: "Between these pages is a wild sea raging, uncontrollably. Its enormous waves engulfing me in tortured silence that no language can describe."[152] Caseness would tend to erase those silences or describe them as a void. But a Narrative view might compare this silence to what Crites calls "sacred stories," stories too deep to be told, where the "story itself creates a world of consciousness."[153]

Since people sometimes exaggerate and project their anger, the question can be raised as to the reliability of the narrator. R.C. Allen even refers to "narrational frenzy," a frantic attempt to find identity by making up stories.[154] But the Caseness approach, also dependent on self-report, is inherently liable to distortion and incompleteness. If people are told that their mind is imbalanced, would it not undermine their confidence? If forced treatment or pressured treatment is in the air, would not one circumscribe his or her own self report? And memory, essential to constructing one's story, may be impaired by psychiatric drugs. Rarely do professionals admit this, as does the psychoanalyst Alice Miller, who wrote that psychiatrists "employ dangerous drugs to destroy the very thing that has potential to heal him: namely, his memory."[155] Recent research suggests that "dopamine down-regulation" by neuroleptic drugs has "especially profound effects on working memory."[156] Literature that advocates for expanded use of shock treatment refers to its "profound memory disturbances."[157] Ironically, ECT advocates cite studies that permanent damage is confined to "a subset of patients who subjectively complained about their memory."[158]

Rather than establishing a new ownership and power disparity, as in Caseness, the Narrative approach encourages respect for the other as a full partner. From doctors or therapists who possess the truth in a monologic fashion, we move toward descriptions such as "ritual companionship," a term used to describe the initiate's guide in indigenous cultures.[159] Kierkegaard identifies the key element of such a companion as one who participates in the other's suffering, such that "it is his own case that is in question."[160] Morson and Emerson explore Bakhtin's dialogic conception of the truth, one that allows other voices "the direct power to mean."[161] By its very nature, the story invites us to enter into the lived world of the other. Such involvement entails imagination, exposure to one's own pain and joy, as well as a willingness to be involved with the mundane needs of the other, traits from which professionalism may seek to distance itself.

Admittedly, there is a risk of being submerged in another's story, slipping into "raw romanticism," as McHugh would say.[162] But it is only by entering into another's story, while maintaining one's own identity, that a true dialogue can ensue.

After taking a narrative of a person's life story, I find that a unique bond is established. The one who tells the story grows in stature and becomes an equal. The feeling of connectedness to a ritual companion can become the way in which the person reintegrates into society, in some cases, as a prophetic witness. When a person goes through his or her "breakdown" experience and names it with the support of a ritual companion, a dynamic for change is released. This leads us to our third and final consideration.

III. Supporting the Transformative Power of Story

A transformative impact usually follows the allowing of the story, telling the narrative, as well as its publication. May refers to a "Phoenix" effect - a new self rising from the ashes of a traumatic physical illness.[163] Frank believes that "At the core of any illness narrative is an epiphany."[164]

There has long been a key assumption in the Narrative approach: that healing imagery arises during periods of deep psychological distress.[165] For Joe Green it was the "lower frequencies of the earth." For Jack it was "a flowing and milky type of energy."[166]

Symbols work, in part, because they mediate pain, as opposed to encouraging a flight from pain. This function can be made clearer with an example from my own "symbolic experience," when I was 18 years old. My psychiatrist believed that periods of turmoil were necessary for growth to occur. Likewise, he believed that he should "support the disorganization," and did not prescribe psychiatric drugs or shock treatment. Here is a vignette from my own experience, first citing the nursing report in my medical record.

> *1:35 P.M. Patient assisted out of bed and told to walk to the end of the hall and sit down to write his thoughts on the pad. Patient very slowly staggered to the table at end of the hall, but did not write anything.*

This note did not begin to capture my inner experience:

> *At the last safe table in the universe, I'm pushed and placed into the last safe chair. The whole universe has changed into this hard, square table of suffering wood. I place my hands on it, then take them away, for it only makes the pain worse. Somehow, I'm already on the inside. When will I join them in pain? On the table I spy a crumpled piece of metal. Is this what I've done to my friend? The Savior's been forced through the Hitler Machine's endless fire and grinding. Is this all that's left of him? A bit of metal, I can barely see glimmer?*

In the midst of this painful and seemingly paranoid delusion, there emerged a symbol of hope. The "bit of metal" was experienced as a spiritual presence small enough to reach me in my pit of despair. Fragmented like myself, it became my invisible ritual companion.

Manifold interpretations of this symbolism are possible. A Jungian might hold that the table represented a mandala of the self, with the bit of metal as its center. Schafer might describe such "pathological signs" as "bits and pieces of the shattered self trying to protect itself, heal itself, and continue its growth."[167] A theologian might interpret it as a call for our society to find spirituality in the most disguised and rejected of forms.[168] But in the Caseness system, a patient who sits and stares at a bit of metal exhibits only a "negative sign" of schizophrenia.

Perhaps an essential transformative effect of going through the "psychotic process" is that the person becomes more feeling oriented, as Jack did after his melting. John Weir says that after the old self dies off, "the warmth is there, the trust relationship, the lovingness. And that's really the fruit of this whole process."[169] In a recent study, compared a number of ex-patients and found that those who had crisis episodes with more florid symptoms came to a higher level of functioning with a greater affective awareness.[170]

If the story is allowed, there follows the transformative effect engendered by its telling. Broyard suggests that it is natural for a person who has a physical illness to "make a story, a narrative, out of his illness as a way of trying to detoxify it."[171] Insofar as the essence of madness is silence, narrative offers an antidote. In dealing with the tension between one's "heroic madness" and a deflationary telling, Felman suggests that the more balanced identity emerges through a process of revision.[172] And if there is a corrective "shrinking," then there can also be a corrective expansion, where "desire is wrought" out of a "narrative web." According to Rushdy, it is not thought or reflection that awakens love within us, but rather the stories we share with each other.[173]

The telling of the narrative has an integrative effect.[174] As Jack explained, "Instead of it going round and round your head, it becomes a part of you."[175] In part, it happens as the "shadow side" of the self which has been invisible comes into view. In part this happens through the validation of the story by another.

There remains the transformative impact of the act of publishing narratives. Giving the person's story the dignity of print radically empowers the individual. People in our culture recognize the power of the printed word, and may read with compassion what they would not believe if it were only spoken. The narrative also reveals the abuses that are perpetrated against the story's protagonist. In an anthology, the repeated pattern of stories shows that a dark side of the mental health system exists and cannot be explained away as paranoid ideation. Because of the validation offered by making public one's account of suffering, the person finds his or her status markedly enhanced.

A published narrative helps people "find their own tribe," as an ex-patient, Josie K., stated.[176] An anthology allows others to realize they are not alone in their suffering. Part of "craziness" is feeling that no one else compares to you. Campbell refers to testimony as "a primary means by which clients transform themselves from marginalized, isolated victims to historical subjects and members of a vital subculture."[177] This feeling of connectedness extends to the cosmological. After the publication of his story, Josie dreamt that he was a giant who climbed to the top of a mesa, and reached out and touched the sky.[178]

SUMMARY AND CONCLUSION

In this paper I have suggested that the life story or Narrative approach is a far more fruitful construct than the Caseness approach. In *Schizophrenia as a Life Style*, Burton defines "schizophrenia" as a thwarting of one's life story.[179] It is when one's story has been stopped that the person becomes "crazy." Thus, symptoms become expressions or cries against that stoppage, which tends to have its roots in the past, sometimes going back to childhood. If the psyche possesses a natural movement toward healing, we may expect to find the way out of "psychosis" encoded in the symptoms.

This article has shown narrative to be a useful tool for understanding the complex phenomena called schizophrenia, within a frame of reference that allows it as a potentially transformative experience. Narrative is robust in its ability to pick up detail while at the same time establishing connections, making for a narrative unity and truth. Highlighting change helps the person refuse "schizophrenia" as a fixed state, and view it instead as a process or passage. A narrative calls forth one's moral responsibility with the self as an active agent, traits important for change. Narrative dignifies one's communication to the larger society, exposing realities which are not usually allowed expression. In contrast, the Caseness approach tends to fix the "schizophrenic" process. It "chronicalizes" the person by establishing a monologic discourse with a predetermined meaning, and thus elicits passivity and compliance. Any value in the experience is discredited.

Ultimately, whether one chooses the Caseness or Narrative approach as the guidepost to understanding the psychiatrically labeled, is an expression of a deep-seated philosophy. If our goal is to control, manage, or shut down expressions of deep suffering, the Caseness approach is sufficient. If, on the other hand, we see something of potential value in the "breakdown" experience for the person and for ourselves, the Narrative approach can serve as our frame of reference.

If symptom control is our ultimate standard, we may be willing to condemn people to half-lives and quarter-lives, in which individuals may lose that creative edge and dynamism that enable them to make a valued social contribution. In the context of a life story, this choice represents a marked diminution or a premature end. If the Narrative approach is our touchstone, the qualitative measure, the richness of a person's life, is our concern. We will be judged by how we become a part of this story, whether we have thwarted the person's life story, or allowed it to deepen and blossom.

References

Adams, C.L. (2020). *Psychosis and the Humpty-Dumpty Story: Dr. Adams' Treatment Philosophy.* AllrOneofUs Publishing.

Alcoff, L., and Gray, L., (1993). Survivor discourse: Transgression or recuperation? Signs: *Journal of Women in Culture and Society* 18, 260-290.

Allen, B. (1985). In the thick of things: Texture in orally communicated history. *International Journal of Oral History* 6, 92-103.

Allen, R.C. (1993). When narrative fails. *Journal of Religious Ethics* 21, 27-67.

American Psychiatric Association. (1994). *Diagnostic and Statistical Manual of Mental Disorders* (fourth edition). Washington, D.C.: Author.

Artin, T. (1974). *The Allegory of Adventure: Reading Chretien's Eric and Yvain.* London: Bucknell University Press.

Balakian, P. (1989). *Theodore Roethke's Far Fields: The Evolution of His Poetry.* Baton Rouge and London: Louisiana State University Press.

Baldessarini, R.J. [Speaker]. (1990, November). Update on antipsychotic agents and treatment of psychiatric disorders. (Cassette Recording No. IA). The Sheppard Pratt National Symposium on Schizophrenia, Baltimore, Maryland.

Balint, E. (1968). *The Basic Fault: Therapeutic Aspects of Regression.* London: Tavistock.

Barrett, R.J. (1988). Clinical writings and the documentary construction of schizophrenia. *Culture, Medicine, and Psychiatry* 12, 265-299.

Barros, C.A. (1992). Figura, persona, dynamis: Autobiography and change. *Biography*, 15, 1-28.

Bayley, C. (1993). Homeopathy. *The Journal of Medicine and Philosophy* 18, 129-145.

Bentall, R. (1990). The syndromes and symptoms of psychosis: Or why you can't play "twenty questions" with the concept of schizophrenia and hope to win. In R. Bentall (Ed.), *Restructuring Schizophrenia* (pp. 23-60). London: Routledge.

Bleuler, M. (1972). The genesis and nature of schizophrenia. In G. Usdin (Ed.), *The Psychiatric*

Forum (pp. 3-15). New York: Brunner/Mazel, Inc.

Bowes, H.A. (1958). The ataractic drugs: The present position of Chlorpromazine, Frenquel, Pacatal, and Reserpine in the psychiatric hospital. In H.L. Gordon (Ed.), *The New Chemotherapy* (pp. 10-22). New York: Philosophical Library.

Breggin, P.R. (1991). *Toxic Psychiatry: Why therapy, empathy, and love must replace the drugs, electroshock, and biochemical theories of the new psychiatry*. New York: St. Martin's Press.

Bromberg, P.M. (1991). On knowing one's patient's inside out: The aesthetics of unconscious communication. Psychoanalytic Dialogues: *A Journal of Relational Perspectives* 1, 399-422.

Broyard, A. (1992). *Intoxicated by My Illness and Other Writings on Life and Death*. New York: Ballantine Books.

Buckley T., and Gottlieb, A. (1988). A critical appraisal of theories of menstrual symbolism. In T. Buckley and A. Gottlieb (Eds.), *Blood Magic: The Anthropology of Menstruation* (pp. 3-50). Berkeley and Los Angeles, California: University of California Press.

Burnham, D.L. (1984). Symbolic vessels for voyages of self-cure. *Psychiatry*, 47, 18-27.

Burnham, D.L. (1993, June). Introduction for The interface between neurobiology and psychodynamics. Symposium conducted by the Washington Psychoanalytic Foundation, the Washington School of Psychiatry. Bethesda, Maryland.

Burstow, B., and Weitz, D. (Eds.). (1988). *Shrink Resistant: The struggle against psychiatry in Canada*. Vancouver, British Columbia: New Star Books.

Burton, A. (1974). *The Alchemy of Schizophrenia*. In A. Burton (Ed.), Schizophrenia as a life style (pp. 36-105). New York: Springer Publishing Company.

Bynum, C. W. (1991). *Fragmentation and Redemption: Essays on Gender and the Human Body in Medieval Religion*. New York: Zone Books.

Calev A., Pass, H.L., Shapira, B., Fink, M., Tubi, N., and Lerer, B. (1993). ECT and memory. In C.E. Coffey (Ed.), *The Clinical Science of Electroconvulsive Therapy* (pp. 125-142). Washington, D.C.: American Psychiatric Press.

Campbell, J. (1991). *Towards Undiscovered Country: Mental health clients speak for themselves*. Unpublished doctoral dissertation, University of California, Irvine.

Canguilhem, G. (1978). *The Normal and the Pathological* [C.R. Fawcett, Trans.]. New York: Zone Books. (Original work published 1966)

Cassell, E. (1985). *Talking with Patients*. Cambridge: MIT Press.

Caussade, J.P. (1987). *Self Abandonment to Divine Providence* [A. Thorold, Trans.]. Rockford, Illinois: Tan Books and Publishers. (Original work published 1861.)

Chadwick, W. (1991). El mundo magico: Lenora Carrington's enchanted garden. In P. Draher (Ed.), *Lenora Carrington: The Mexican Years* (pp. 9-31). San Francisco: The Mexican Museum.

Charon, R. (1992). To build a case: Medical histories as traditions in conflict. *Literature and Medicine*, 11, 115-132.

Charon, R. (1993). Medical interpretation: Implications of literary theory of narrative for clinical work. *Journal of Narrative and Life History* 3, 79-97.

Corin, E., and Lauzon, G. (1992). Positive withdrawal and the quest for meaning: The reconstruction of experience among schizophrenics. *Psychiatry* 55, 266-278.

Couser, G.T. (1991). *Autopathography: Women, Illness, and Lifewriting*. a/b: Auto/biography studies, 6, 65-75.

Crammer, J. (1990). *Asylum History*: Buckinghamshire County Pauper Lunatic Asylum -St. John's. London: Gaskell.

Crites, S. (1989). The narrative quality of experience. In S. Hauerwas and L.G. Jones (Eds.), *Why Narrative? Readings in narrative theology* (pp. 65-88). Grand Rapids, Michigan: William B. Eerdmans Publishing Company.

Doherry, E.G. (1975). Labelling effects in psychiatric hospitalization: A study of diverging patterns of inpatient self-labelling processes. *Archives of General Psychiatry* 32, 562-568.

Dulcan, M.K. (1990). Using psychostimulants to treat behavioral disorders of children and adolescents. *Journal of Child and Adolescent Psychopharmacology* I, 7-20.

Eliade, M. (1958). *Rites and Symbols of Initiation: The Mysteries of Birth and Rebirth* [W.R. Trask, Trans.]. New York: Harper and Row Publishers.

Eliade, M. (1991). *Images and Symbols* [P. Mairet, Trans.]. Princeton, New Jersey: Princeton University Press. (Original work published 1952)

Estroff, S.E. (1992). Everybody's got a little mental illness: Accounts of illness and self among people with severe, persistent mental illnesses. *Medical Anthropology Quarterly* 5, 331-369.

Farher, S. (1993). [Interview with Leonard Frank]. *Madness, Heresy and the Rumor of Angels*. Chicago and LaSalle, Illinois: Open Court.

Felman, S. (1985). *Writing and Madness*: (Literature/philosophy/psychoanalysis) [M.N. Evans, Trans.]. Ithaca, New York: Cornell University Press. (Original work published 1978)

Fichtelberg, J. (1989). *The Complex Image: Faith and Method in American Autobiography*. Philadelphia: University of Pennsylvania Press.

Fishbein, M. (1958). The tranquillizing drugs. In H.L. Gordon (Ed.), *The New Chemotherapy* (pp. 3-6). New York: Philosophical Library.

Fleischmann, N. (1988). Journal. In B. Burstow and D. Weitz (Eds.), *Shrink Resistant. The Struggle Against Psychiatry in Canada* (pp. 80-86). Vancouver, British Columbia: New Star Books.

Frank, AW. (1993). The rhetoric of self-change: Illness experience as narrative. *The Sociological Quarterly* 34 39-52.

Frankl, V.E. (1986). *The Doctor and the Soul: From psychotherapy to logotherapy* (revised edition) [R. and C. Winston, Trans.]. New York: Vintage Books. (Original work published 1952)

Goldwert, M. (1992). The psychiatrist as shaman: Sullivan and schizophrenia. *Psychological Reports* 70 669-670.

Good, G. (1992). Identity and form in the modem autobiographical essay. *Prose Studies* 15, 99-117.

Gordon, H.L. (Ed.). (1958). *The New Chemotherapy in Mental Illness: The History, Pharmacology and Clinical Experiences with Rauwolfia, Phenothiazine, Azacyclonol, Mephenesin, Hydroxyzine and Benactyzine preparations*. New York: Philosophic Library Inc.

Gordon, J.S. (1993, September). The integration of mind and body approaches in practice. Paper presented at Mental health practice in the nineties: Changes and challenges, A Conference in honor of Loren Mosher, M.D., Silver Spring, Maryland.

Grof, S. (1976). *Realms of the Human Unconscious: Observations from LSD Research*. New York: E.P. Dutton.

Grof, S. (1992). *The Holotopic Mind: The Three Levels of Human Consciousness and How They Shape Our Lives*. New York: Harper San Francisco, A Division of Harper Collins Publishers.

Hall, J.A. (1987). Personal transformation: The inner image of initiation. In L.C. Mahdi, S. Foster, and M. Little (Eds.), *Betwixt and Between: Patterns of masculine and feminine initiation* (pp. 327-337). Peru, Illinois: Open Court.

Hall, L.L. (Ed.). (1992). *The Biology of Mental Disorders: New developments in neuroscience* (Report No. OTA-BA-538). Washington D.C.: U.S. Congress, Office of Technology Assessment.

Hallstein, A.L. (1992). Spiritual opportunities in the liminal rites of hospitalization. *Journal of Religion and Health* 31, 247-254.

Hermans, H., Rijks, T., and Kempen, H. (1993). Imaginal dialogues in the self: Theory and method. *Journal of Personality* 61, 207-236.

Hill, S., and Goodwin, J.R. (1993). Demonic possession as a consequence of childhood trauma. *The Journal of Psychohistory* 20, 399-411.

Hoffman, E.R., and McGlashan, T.H. (1993). Neurodynamics and schizophrenia research: Editor's Introduction. *Schizophrenia Bulletin* 19, 15-19.

Hoffman, L. (1981). *Foundations of Family Therapy: A Conceptual Framework for Systems Change*. New York: Basic Books.

Hubbard, R., and Wald, E. (1993). *Exploding the Gene Myth: How genetic information is produced and manipulated by scientists, physicians .employers, insurance companies, educators. and law enforcers*. Boston, Massachusetts: Beacon Press.

Hugh-Jones, S. (1979). *The Palm and the Pleiades: Initiation and cosmology in northwest Amazonia*. Cambridge, England: Cambridge University Press.

Jackson, S. W. (1990). The use of passions in psychological healing. *Journal of the History of Medicine* 45, 150-175.

Jung, C.G. (1991). *Psyche and Symbol* (R.F. Hull, Trans.). Princeton, New Jersey: Princeton University Press. (Original work published 1958)

Kaam, A., and Healy, K. (1967). *The Demon and the Dove: Personality Growth Through Literature*. Pittsburgh: Duquesne University Press.

Kalinowsky, L.B. (1958) Chlorpromazine and reserpine, and their relation to other treatments in psychiatry. In H.L. Gordon (Ed.), *The New Chemotherapy* (pp. 343-350). New York: Philosophical Library.

Kane, J.M. (1990). Psychopharmacologic treatment of schizophrenia. In A. Kales, C. Stefanis, and J. Talbott (Eds.), *Recent Advances in Schizophrenia* (pp. 257-276). New York: Springer-Verlag.

Kierkegaard, S. (1980). *The Concept of Anxiety: A simple psychologically orienting deliberation on the dogmatic issue of hereditary sin* (R. Thomte, Trans.). Princeton, New Jersey: Princeton University Press. (Original work published 1844)

Kinross-Wright, V. (1958). Chlorpromazine treatment of mental disorders. In H.L. Gordon (Ed.), *The New Chemotherapy* (pp. 292-299). New York: Philosophical Library.

Kirmayer, L.J. (1992). The body's insistence on meaning: Metaphor as presentation and representation in illness experience. *Medical Anthropology Quarterly* 6, 323-346.

Kuhl, V. (1994). The managed care revolution: Implications for humanistic psychotherapy. *Journal of Humanistic Psychology* 34, 62-81.

Landau, E.G. (1989). *Jackson Pollock*. New York: Harry N. Abrams, Inc.

Lattas, M. (1992). Hysteria, anthropological disclosure and the concept of the unconscious: Cargo cults and the scientization of race and colonial power. *Oceania*, 63, 1-15.

Lecuona, J., Joseph, K., Iqbal N., and Asnis, G. (1993). Dopamine hypothesis of schizophrenia revisited. *Psychiatric Annals* 23, 179-185.

Leff, J. (1991). Schizophrenia in the melting pot. *Nature*, 353, 693-694.

Lewis-Fernandez, R., and Kleinman, A. (1994). Culture, personality, and psychopathology. *Journal of Abnormal Psychology*, 103, 67-71.

Lucksted, A., and Coursey, R.D. (1992). *Consumer perceptions of pressure and force in psychiatric treatments*. Master's thesis, University of Maryland, College Park.

Lukoff, D., Turner R., and Lu, F. (1992). Transpersonal psychology research review. Psycho-religious dimensions of healing. Journal of Transpersonal Psychology, 24, 41-60.

Lux, K. E. (1976). A mystical-occult approach to psychosis. In P.A. Magaro (Ed.), *The Construction of Madness: Emerging Conceptions and Interventions* (pp. 93-132). New York: Pergamon Press Inc.

MacGregor, J .M. (1989). *The Discovery of the Art of the Insane.* Princeton, New Jersey: Princeton University Press.

Maine, D.R. (1993). Narrative's moment and sociology's phenomena: Toward a narrative sociology. *The Sociological Quarterly* 34, 17-38.

Martensson, L. (1991, Autumn). The meaning of life effaced: The impact of neuroleptics. *The Rights Tenet* (Newsletter of the National Association for Rights Protection and Advocacy), pp.4-5.

Martin, P.A. (1972). Obnoxiousness in psychiatric patients and others. In G. Usdin (Ed.), *The Psychiatric Forum* (pp. 59-65). New York: Brunner/Mazel, Inc.

Mason, M.J. (1993). Re-visioning clients' pathology into initiatory desire. *Counseling and Values* 38, 4-11.

Masson, J.M. (1991). *Final Analysis: The making and unmaking of a psychoanalyst.* New York: Harper Perennial.

May, W.F. (1991). *The Patient's Ordeal.* Bloomington, Indiana: Indiana University Press.

McGlashan, T.H. (1993). Schizophrenia: The evolution from psychodynamics to neurodynamics. Paper presented at The interface between neurobiology and psychodynamics. Symposium conducted by the Washington Psychoanalytic Foundation, The Washington School of Psychiatry, Bethesda, Maryland.

McHugh, P.R. (1994, Winter). Psychotherapy awry. *The American Scholar* p. 17-30.

McHugh, P.R., and Slavney, P.R. (1986). *The Perspectives of Psychiatry.* Baltimore: Johns Hopkins University Press.

Mendel, W.M. (1976). *Schizophrenia: The Experience and its Treatment.* San Francisco and London: Jossey-Bass Publishers.

Miller, A. (1991). *Breaking Down the Wall of Silence: The Liberating Experience of Facing Painful Truth* (S. Worral, Trans.). New York: Dutton.

Miller, J. (1990). Mental illness and spiritual crisis: Implications for psychiatric rehabilitation. *Psychosocial Rehabilitation Journal* 14, 29-47.

Mochulsky, K. (1970). Dostoevsky and the brothers Karamazov [M.A. Minihan, Trans.]. Introduction in F. Dostoevsky, *The Brothers Karamazov*. New York: Bantam Books Inc.

Monroe, R.R. (1992). *Creative Brainstorms: The Relationship Between Madness and Genius*. New York: Irvington Publishers, Inc.

Moore, T. (1990). *The Planets Within: The Astrological Psychology of Marsilio Ficino*. Hudson, New York: Lindisfarne Press.

Morgenthaler, W. (1992). *Madness and Art: The Life and Works of Adolf Wolfi*. Lincoln and London: University of Nebraska Press.

Morson, U.S., & Emerson, C. (1990). *Mikhail Bakhtin: Creation of a Prosaics*. Stanford, California: Stanford University Press.

Mount, E. (1993). Can we talk? Contexts of meaning for interpreting illness. *The Journal of Medical Humanities* 14, 51-65.

Mowaljarlai, D., and Malnic, J. (1993). *Yorro Yorro: Aboriginal creation and the renewal of nature*. Rochester, Vermont: Inner Traditions.

Nixon, R. (1993). Of Balkans and Bantustans: AEthnic cleansing(and the crisis in national legitimation. *Transitions: An International Review* 60, 4-26.

Noble, R.C. (1993). Physicians and the pharmaceutical industry: An alliance with unhealthy aspects. *Perspectives in Biology and Medicine* 36, 376-394.

Nobler, M.S., and Sackeim, H.A. (1993). ECT stimulus dosing: Relations to efficacy and adverse effects. In C.E. Coffey (Ed.), *The Clinical Science of Electroconvulsive Therapy* (pp. 29-52). Washington, D.C.: American Psychiatric Press.

Oakes, J.G.H. (Ed.). (1991). *In the Realms of the Unreal: "Insane" Writings*. New York: Four Walls Eight Windows.

O'Mara, R. (1994, March 11). Balkan war pushes one Baltimore woman into unilateral action. *The Baltimore Sun*, pp. Dl, D2.

Ortolf, D. (1994). *The classical, mystical experience and alexithymia in advanced spiritual practitioners and renewal process psychoses.* Doctoral dissertation, United States International University, San Diego, California.

Peck, M. (1978). *The Road Less Traveled: A New Psychology of Love, Traditional Values and Spiritual Growth.* New York: Simon and Schuster.

Perry, J. W. (1987). *The Self in Psychotic Process: Its Symbolization in Schizophrenia* (revised edition). Dallas, Texas: Spring Publications. (Original work published 1953)

Perry, J.W. (1990). Visionary experience or psychosis. In *Thinking Allowed: Conversations on the leading edge of knowledge and discovery with Dr. Jeffrey Mishlove* (pp. 1-10). [Available from: Institute of Noetic Sciences. 475 Gate 5 Road, Suite 300, Sausalito, California 94966.]

Pert, C.B. (1993, September). The integration of endorphins and environment on mental Status. Paper presented at *Mental Health Practice in the Nineties: Changes and Challenges*, A Conference in Honor of Loren Mosher, M.D., Silver Spring, Maryland.

Pickar, D. (Speaker). (1990, November). Improving response with novel psychotropics. (Cassette Recording No. IB). Paper presented at The Sheppard Pratt National Symposium on Schizophrenia, Baltimore, Maryland.

Pinel, P. (1983). *A Treatise on Insanity: In which are contained the principles of a new and more practical nosology of maniacal disorders* [D.D. Davis, Trans.]. Birmingham, Alabama: Gryphon Editions, Ltd. (Original work published 1806)

Pinheiro, M.V. (1992). The selling of clinical psychiatry in America. *Hospital and Community Psychiatry*, 43, 102-104.

Pious, W.L. (1961). A Hypothesis About the Nature of Schizophrenic Behavior. In A. Burton (Ed.), *Psychotherapy of the Psychosis* (pp. 43-68). New York: Basic Books.

Podvoll, E.M. (1990) .*The Seduction of Madness: Revolutionary Insights into the World of Psychosis and a Compassionate Approach to Recovery at Home.* New York: Harper Collins Publishers.

Risse, G.B., and Warner, J .H. (1992). Reconstructing clinical activities: Patient records in medical history. *Social History of Medicine*, 5, 183-205.

Rodgers, J.E. (1992). *Psychosurgery: Damaging the brain to save the mind.* New York: Harper Collins. Rose, S.M. (1991). Another unveiling: Abuse backgrounds of psychiatric survivors and their neglect by mental health systems. In M.A. Susko (Ed.), *Cry of the invisible* (pp. 317-320). Baltimore, Maryland: The Conservatory Press.

Rushdy, A.H.A. (1993). Cartesian mirror/Quixotic web: Toward a narrativity of desire. *Mosaic*, 26, 83-110.

Saraceno, B., Tognoni, G., and Garattini, S. (1993). Critical questions in clinical psychopharmacology. In N. Sartorius, G. Girolamo, G. Andrews, G.A. German, and L. Eisenberg (Eds.), *Treatment of Mental Disorders: A Review of Effectiveness* (pp. 63-90). Washington, D.C.: American Psychiatric Press.

Sarbin, T.R. (1990). Toward the obsolescence of the schizophrenia hypothesis. *The Journal of Mind and Behavior*, 11, 259-283.

Sass, L.A. (1992a). Heidegger, schizophrenia and the ontological difference. *Philosophical Psychology*, 5, 109-132.

Sass, L.A. (1992b). *Madness and Modernism: Insanity in the Light of Art, Literature, and Thought.* New York: Basic Books.

Scarry, E. (1985). *The Body in Pain: The Making and Unmaking of the World.* New York and Oxford: Oxford University Press.

Schafer, R. (1983). *The Analytic Attitude.* New York: Basic Books.

Scheff, T.J. (1979). *Catharsis in Healing, Ritual and Drama.* Berkeley: University of California Press.

Scull, A. (1991). Psychiatry and social control in the nineteenth and twentieth centuries. *History of Psychiatry*, 2, 149-169.

Sechehaye, M.A. (1951). *Symbolic Realization: A New Method of Psychotherapy Applied to a Case of Schizophrenia* [B. Wursten and H. Wursten Trans.]. New York: International Universities Press, Inc.

Showalter, E. (1993). On hysterical narrative. *Narrative*, 1, 24-35.

Silverman, J. (1967). Shamanism and acute schizophrenia. *American Anthropologist*, 69, 21-31.

Smith, D.H. (1993). Stories, values and patient care decisions. In C. Conrad (Ed.), *The Ethical Nexus* (pp. 123-148). Norwood, New Jersey: Ablex Publishing.

Spaniol, L., and Koehler M. (1994). The experience of recovery. [Available from The Center for Psychiatric Rehabilitation, Sargent College of Allied Health Professions, Boston University, 730 Commonwealth Avenue, Boston, Massachusetts 02215.]

Spiegel, D. (Ed.). (1993). *Dissociative Disorders: A Clinical Review*. Baltimore, Maryland: Sidran Press.

Spohn, H.E., Coyne, L., Larson, J., Mittleman, F., Spray, J., and Hayes, K. (1986). Episodic and residual thought pathology in chronic schizophrenics: Effect of neuroleptics. *Schizophrenic Bulletin*, 12, 394-407.

Stone, M.H. (1993). *Abnormalities of Personality: Within and Beyond the Realm of Treatment*. New York: W.W. Norton.

Strassman, R.J. (1991) Human hallucinogenic drug research in the United States: A present-day case history and review of the process. *Journal of Psychoactive Drugs*, 23, 29-38.

Striano, J. (1988). *Can Psychotherapists Hurt You!* Santa Barbara, California: Professional Press.

Sullivan, L.E. (1988). *lcanthus Drum: An orientation to meaning in South American religions*. New York: MacMillan Publishing Co.

Sullivan, L.E. (1993, Spring). Images of wholeness: Interview with Lawrence E. Sullivan. *Parabola. The Magazine of Myth and Tradition*, 8, 4-13.

Susko, M.A. (Ed.). (1991). *Cry of the Invisible*: *Writings from the Homeless and Psychiatric Survivors*. Baltimore, Maryland: The Conservatory Press.

Susko, M.A. (1993). The APA convention and counter convention. Disability Studies Quarterly, 13,8-11.

Szasz, T. (1993). Crazy talk: Thought disorder or psychiatric arrogance? *British Journal of Medical Psychology*, 66, 61-67.

Thieves, M. (1992, Summer). Art and psychosis. *Raw Vision: International Journal of Intuitive and Visionary Art,* pp. 34-39.

Thompson, R. (1993, September). The Iron Triangle. Paper presented at *Mental Health Practice in the Nineties: Changes and Challenges, A Conference in honor of Loren Mosher, M.D.*, Silver Spring, Maryland.

Tirrell, L. (1990). Storytelling and moral agency. *The Journal of Aesthetics and Art Criticism*, 48, 115-126.

Torrey, E.F. (1972). *The Mind Game: Witchdoctors and Psychiatrists*. New York: Bantam Books. Treichler, P.A. (1992). Escaping the sentence: Diagnosis and discourse in "The Yellow

Wallpaper." (In C. Golden (Ed.), *The Captive Imagination: A Casebook on The Yellow Wallpaper* (pp. 191-210). New York: The Feminist Press at The City University of New York.

Ussher, J. (1991). *Women's Madness: Misogyny or Mental Illness*. Amherst, Massachusetts: The University of Massachusetts Press.

Vitz, P.C. (1992). Narratives and counseling, Part I: From analysis of the past to stories about it. *Journal of Psychology and Theology*, 20, 11-19.

Wakefield, J.C. (1992). Disorder as harmful dysfunction: A conceptual critique of DSM-III-R's definition of mental disorder. *Psychological Review*, 99, 232-247.

Weiss, K.M. (1992). On the distinctions between diagnosis, description and measurement of schizophrenia. *Psychopathology*, 25, 239-248.

Wikler, D., and Barondess, J. (1993). Bioethics and anti-bioethics in light of Nazi medicine: What must we remember? *Kennedy Institute of Ethics Journal*, 3, 39-55.

Williams, J.G. (1991). *The Bible, Violence and the Sacred: Liberation from the Myth of Sanctioned Violence.* New York: Harper Collins Publishers.

Willick, M.S. (1993). The deficit syndrome in schizophrenia: Psychoanalytic and neurobiological perspectives. *Journal of the American Psychoanalytic Association*, 41, 1135-1157.

Wilson, M. (1993). DSM-III and the transformation of American psychiatry: A history. *The American Journal of Psychiatry,* 150, 399-410.

Zoja, L. (1989). *Drugs, Addiction and Initiation: The Modern Search for Ritual.* Boston: Sigo Press.

Endnotes

[1]. See Burstow and Weitz, 1988; Oakes, 1991; Spaniol and Koehler, 1994; Susko, 1991).

[2]. Miller, 1991

[3]. Risse and Warner, 1992

[4]. See Canguilhem, 1966/1978. p. 192.

[5]. See Cassell, 1985.

[6]. Broyard, 1992 p. 18.

[7]. Charon, 1992.

[8]. Sullivan, 1993, p. 6.

[9]. Bynum, 1991.

[10]. Bayley, 1993.

[11]. Frank, cited in Farber, 1993.

[12]. Crammer, 1990, p. 11.

[13]. Smith, 1993, p. 128

[14]. Pert, 1993.

[15]. Jung 1958/1991 p. 147.

[16]. Personal communication, September 1993.

[17]. Mowaljarlai and Malnic, 1993, p. 81.

[18]. Lecuona, Joseph, Iqbal, and Asnis, 1993.

[19]. Pickar, 1990.

[20]. Leff, 1991; Weiss, 1992.

[21]. Willick, 1993.

[22]. Szasz, 1993, p. 61.

[23]. Pert, 1993.

[24]. Cited in Susko, 1993.

[25]. Striano, 1988, p. 6.

[26]. Scull, 1991.

[27]. Lattas, 1992, p. 4.

[28]. Miller, 1991.

[29]. Hoffman, 1981.

[30]. Martin, 1972.

[31]. See Stone, 1993.

[32]. Ussher, 1991, p.13.

[33]. Treichler, 1992, p. 195.

[34]. Kuhl, 1994.

[35]. Pinheiro, 1992, p. 102.

[36]. Noble, 1993, p. 380.

[37]. Williams 1991, p. 248.

[38]. Sarbin, 1990; Szasz, 1993.

[39]. Bentall, 1990.

[40]. Weiss, 1992.

[41]. Bentall, 1990.

[42]. McHugh and Slavney, 1986.

[43]. Hall, 1992.

[44]. Mendell, 1976.

[45]. Frankl, 1952/1986.

[46]. Lux, 1976.

[47]. Bleuler, 1972.

[48]. McGlashan, 1993.

[49]. Barrett, 1988, p. 290.

[50]. Rodgers, 1992.

[51]. Personal communication, June 1993.

[52]. See Morgenthaler, 1992, plate 21; MacGregor, 1989, plate 13.

[53]. Torrey, 1972.

[54]. Hubbard and Wald, 1993, p. 95.

[55]. Wikler and Barondess, 1993, p. 41.

[56]. Nixon, 1993, p. 6.

[57]. Doherty, 1975.

[58]. R. W. Manderscheid, personal communication, June 8, 1993.

[59]. Dulcan, 1990.

[60]. Nobler and Sackeim, 1993.

[61]. Spohn, Coyne, Larson, Mittleman, Spray, and Hayes, 1986.

[62]. Grof, 1976; Strassman, 1991.

[63]. Bowes, 1958.

[64]. Cited in Susko, 1991, p. 297.

[65]. H.L. Gordon, 1958.

[66]. Kane, 1990; Lecuona, Joseph, Iqbal, and Asnis, 1993.

[67]. Cited in Susko, 1991, p. 156.

[68]. Hill and Goodwin, 1993.

[69]. Peck, 1978.

[70]. Masson, 1991, p. 52.

[71]. Fishbein, 1958; Kalinowsky, 1958; Kinross-Wright, 1958.

[72]. Breggin, 1991; Martensson, 1991; see Saraceno, Tognoni, and Garattini, 1993, table 3-3.

[73]. Cited in Susko, 1991, p. 36.

[74]. Baldessarini, 1990.

[75]. Lucksted and Coursey, 1992.

[76]. Ron Thompson, personal communication, March 12, 1994.

[77]. Mount, 1993, p. 61.

[78]. Good, 1992, p. 102.

[79]. Maine, 1993.

[80]. Charon, 1993.

[81]. See Vitz, 1992.

[82]. See Moore, 1990, p. 98.

[83]. Pinel 1806/1983, p. 42.

[84]. See Miller, 1990.

[85]. Corin and Lauzon, 1992.

[86]. Burnham, 1984.

[87]. J. W. Perry, 1990.

[88]. Kaam and Healy, 1967, p. 63.

[89]. Artin, 1974, p. 216.

[90]. Mochulsky, 1970, p. xvi

[91]. Eliade, 1958, p. xiv.

[92]. Cited in Susko, 1991 p. 50.

[93]. Cited in Susko, 1991 p. 50.

[94]. Eliade, 1952/1991, p. 158.

[95]. Moore, 1990, p. l00.

[96]. Kirmayer, 1992, p. 323.

[97]. See Sullivan, 1988.

[98]. Hugh-Jones, 1979, p. 120.

[99]. Goldwert, 1992; Silverman, 1967.

[100]. Mason, 1993, p. 4.

[101]. Cited in Monroe, 1992, p. 20.

[102]. Pious, 1961 p. 51.

[103]. Grof, 1992.

[104]. Zoja, 1989, p. 58.

[105]. Hallstein, 1992, p. 252.

[106]. Scarry, 1985.

[107]. Scheff, 1979.

[108]. Rose, 1991.

[109]. Bromberg, 1991; Balint, 1968.

[110]. See Spiegel, 1993.

[111]. Edith, personal communication, March 18, 1994.

[112]. See Jackson, 1990.

[113]. Sass, 1992a, p. 109.

[114]. Perry, 1987, p. 16.

[115]. Miller, 1991, p. 33.

[116]. A.W. Frank, 1993.

[117]. Thevoz, 1992.

[118]. Chadwick, 1991; Landau, 1989.

[119]. See O=Mara, 1994.

[120]. Podvoll, 1990.

[121]. Cohen, cited by Burnham, 1993.

[122]. Buckley and Gottlieb, 1988.

[123]. Personal communication, May 11, 1994.

[124]. Maine, 1993, p. 17.

[125]. Estroff, 1992,

[126]. Couser, 1991.

[127]. Showalter, 1993.

[128]. Alcoff and Gray, 1993.

[129]. Fichtelberg, 1989, p. 46.

[130]. Good, 1992, p.102.

[131]. Barros, 1992.

[132]. J.S. Gordon, 1993.

[133]. Allen, 1985.

[134]. Felman, 1978/1985, p. 54.

[135]. Fleischmann, 1988, p. 86.

[136]. Lewis-Fernandez and Kleinman, 1994.

[137]. Hermans, Rijks, and Kempen, 1993.

[138]. Sass, 1992b, p. 131.

[139]. Rushdy, 1993.

[140]. Charon, 1993.

[141]. Vitz, 1992.

[142]. Cited in Susko, 1991 p. 110.

[143]. Sarbin, 1990, p. 280.

[144]. Cited in Susko, 1991, p. 53.

[145]. Tirrel, 1990.

[146]. R.C. Allen 1993.

[147]. Barrett, 1988, p. 281.

[148]. Charon, 1993, p. 95.

[149]. Personal communication, October 1993.

[150]. Cited in Balakian, 1989, p. 34.

[151]. Charon, 1993.

[152]. Fleischmann, 1988, p. 82.

[153]. Crites, 1989, p. 71.

[154]. R.C. Allen, 1993.

[155]. A. Miller, 1991, p. 31.

[156]. Hoffman and McGlashan, 1993, p. 15.

[157]. Nobler and Sackeim, 1993, p. 46.

[158]. Calev, Pass, Shapira, Fink, Tubi, and Lerer, 1993, p. 137.

[159]. Sullivan, 1988.

[160]. Kierkegaard, 1844/1980, p. 120.

[161]. Morson and Emerson, 1990, p. 239.

[162]. McHugh 1994.

[163]. May 1991.

[164]. Frank, 1993, p. 41.

[165]. Sechehaye, 1951.

[166]. Cited in Susko, 1991, p. 49.

[167]. Schafer 1983, p. 217.

[168]. Caussade, 1861/1987, p. 22.

[169]. Perry 1990, p. 6.

[170]. Ortolf, 1994.

[171]. Broyard, 1992, p. 21.

[172]. Felman, 1978/1985.

[173]. Rushdy, 1993, p. 95.

[174]. A. Miller, 1991.

[175]. Personal communication, December 1992.

[176]. Personal communication, March 1992.

[177]. Campbell (1991, p. 369.

[178]. Personal communication, March 1992.

[179]. Burton, 1974.

Did you love *Caseness and Narrative: Contrasting Approaches to People Psychiatrically Labelled*? Then you should read *Transformational Stories: Voices for True Healing in Mental Health*[1] by Michael A. Susko!

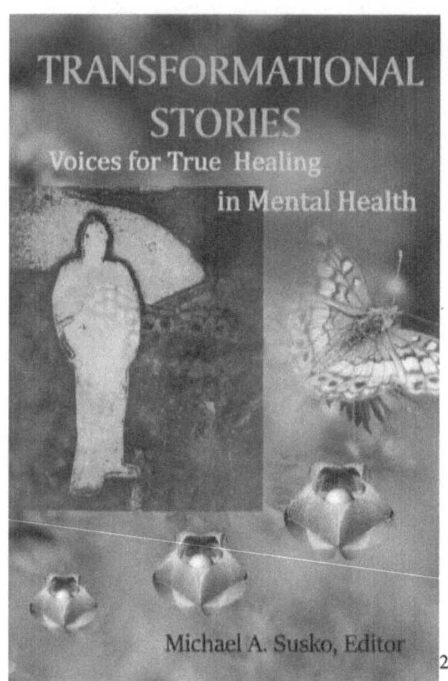

These oral histories tell of transformative experiences which led persons to become advocates and practitioners for reform of the mental health system. They include psychiatric survivors and professionals, many of whom have been or are leaders in the movement. Many of these stories are a miracle of survival, but they show the path to true healing — how, despite fierce resistance, persons found their voice and identity. Pioneered by those who faced extreme situations and wounding, the way to deep healing can be found in lived lifes. We invite you now to take a journey which will convey to you an uncommon psychological wisdom.

Read more at https://www.allroneofus.com/.

---

1. https://books2read.com/u/bzvl09

2. https://books2read.com/u/bzvl09

Also by Michael A. Susko

Archetypal Worlds
Alwon in Another World: An Archetypal Voyage
Line On the Wall
The Alien's Gift
The Gold People
Spider Woman and the Timeroc
Quill Ears & the Other Earth
Darkwood and Dual with the Shadow Side
Giant Under the Mountain

Haikus and Photos
Flowers and Haikus
Haikus and Photos: Guatemalan Highlands
Haikus and Photos: Water Birds and Reflections
Haikus and Photos: Seasons of New River
Haikus and Photos: Yosemite Wilderness
Haikus and Photos: California Coast
Haikus and Photos: Canadian Rockies
Haikus and Photos: Hawaii's Exotic Landscapes
Haikus and Photos: Vienna, People with Buildings and Art
Haikus and Photos: Slovakian Castles and Hamlets
Haikus and Photos: Berlin, Light and Dark

Haikus and Photos: New Orleans, City of Immigrants
Haikus and Photos: Antietam Wind and Spirits

Little Lion
The Lion and the Chameleon
The Elephant and the Chameleons

The Dreaming Series
Sleek Back
Streak and Cave Bear Dreaming
Moby and Marsupial Mole Dreaming

The Dream World Trilogy
Delphi, the Time Thief, and the Dream World
Detinna and the Cave God
The Resistance & the Empire

Worlds to the Side
Down Below and the Archon's Castle
Up Above and the Runaway
Across the Gulf and Journey Into Un-Time
On the Bay and a Child Found
In the Wild and Do One Wild Thing
On the Mountain and Two Are Missing
To the Beginning and Journey Through Here

Watch for more at https://www.allroneofus.com/.

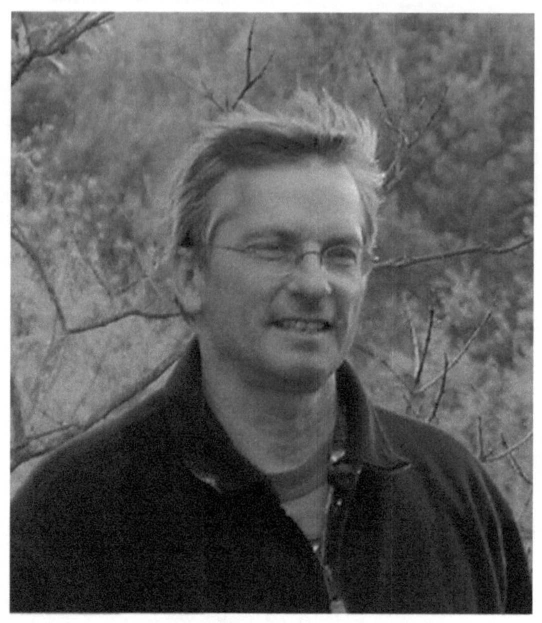

About the Author

Michael Susko, M.S in Counseling Psychology, has been active for several years in advocacy for re-envisioning mental health care. Attending conferences and workshops, he often presented on the meaning of symbolic experiences. In 1991 he edited *Cry of the Invisible*, a collection of oral histories of persons, homeless or psychiatrically labeled. For several years he served on the board for Maryland Disability Rights, to insure the rights of the disabled. The editor has also published works in psychology, evolutionary biology, and creative fiction.

Read more at https://www.allroneofus.com/.